MAGIC OF THE MAYR METHOD

Beginners Guide To The Mayr Method Journey For Health & Wellness

VINCENT JERRY

Table of Contents

Introductory

The Mayr Method, also known as the Mayr Cure or Mayr Therapy, was designed to improve general health and gastrointestinal function.

The technique is based on the premise that gastrointestinal dysfunction and toxic accumulation are at the core of numerous health issues.

The Mayr Method is founded on the following concepts and elements.

- The Mayr Method emphasizes digestive tract detoxification and purification to improve digestion. For this purpose, fasting, calorie restriction, and promoting thorough chewing of food are employed.

• The technique attempts to give the digestive tract a break by consuming fewer solid meals and more easily digestible foods such as broth and herbal teas. This liberates body resources for restoration and repair.

• The Mayr Method promotes healthful eating habits, such as eating slowly, chewing each bite thoroughly, and not going to bed hungry. It promotes eating foods in their natural, unaltered states and avoiding stimulants such as caffeine and alcohol.

• The strategy promotes detoxification via a variety of channels, including the consumption of large volumes of water and herbal teas, as well as targeted therapies such as abdominal massages and hydrotherapy.

• Respect for the individuality of each patient's health care needs is fundamental to the Mayr Method, which promotes individualized treatment approaches.

The objectives of the Mayr Method are to promote digestion, the immune system, energy, weight loss, and overall health. It is a common method of treatment for chronic conditions such as digestive issues, allergies, fatigue, and others.

Always consult your physician before commencing a new therapy or health regimen.

CHAPTER ONE
The Importance Of A Healthy Digestive System

The term "gut health" refers to the condition of the digestive system and its organs, specifically the stomach, intestines, and other associated structures. Gut health is crucial for more than just digestion; it effects an individual's entire body and lifestyle. Among the most persuasive arguments in favor of gastrointestinal health are:

• The digestive tract is responsible for absorbing nutrients from food. Absorption of vitamins, minerals, and macronutrients is essential for good health and appropriate body function, and a healthy gut with optimal digestive function ensures this.

• As much of the immune system is located there, it is beneficial. The microorganisms that reside in our intestines, also known as the gut microbiome, are essential for a healthy immune system.

When the intestinal microbiome is diverse and in balance, the risk of developing auto-immune diseases is reduced, immune responses are strengthened, and dangerous pathogens are thwarted.

• The gut-brain axis is a two-way communication channel between the digestive tract and the brain that plays a crucial role in mental health and mood regulation.

The gastrointestinal microbiome produces neurotransmitters such as serotonin and dopamine, which play a role in mood regulation. Studies have linked dysbiosis in the intestines to psychiatric disorders such as depression and anxiety, as well as neurological disorders such as Alzheimer's and Parkinson's.

• Proper digestion and regular bowel movements: A healthy stomach is essential for the efficient elimination of waste and toxins. Good digestive health prevents constipation, diarrhea, bloating, and irritable bowel syndrome (IBS).

• The condition of a person's digestive tract is directly related to the prevention of inflammation and chronic diseases. Chronic inflammation has been linked to obesity, diabetes, cardiovascular disease, autoimmune disorders, and even some types of cancer. With proper gastrointestinal hygiene, inflammation and the risk of developing chronic diseases can be reduced.

Gut health requires adopting a healthy lifestyle, which includes consuming a balanced diet rich in fiber, prebiotics, and probiotics, engaging in regular physical activity, getting enough sleep, managing stress, and avoiding excessive use of antibiotics and other drugs that may disturb the gut microbiome. Consult a physician if you experience digestive discomfort or if you have concerns about your gastrointestinal health.

Mechanisms Behind The Mayr Diet

The Mayr Diet is a component of the Mayr digestive health and wellness system. The Mayr Method is also known as Mayr Therapy.

These dietary modifications may improve digestion, detoxification, and overall health. How the Mayr Diet typically works:

• On the Mayr Diet, difficult-to-digest or inflammatory foods are typically avoided or consumed in moderation. This category includes substances such as caffeine, caffeine, gluten, dairy products, and refined carbohydrates. The purpose of the diet is to enhance gut health by decreasing the body's digestive stress response by removing these potential causes.

• The Mayr diet encourages consuming foods in their natural, unaltered states because they are easier on the digestive tract. It encourages the consumption of more plant-based foods, such as fruits and vegetables, whole grains, lean meats, and healthful fats. These nutrient-dense foods contain vitamins, minerals, antioxidants, and fiber, all of which promote digestive health and general well-being.

• Conscious eating and thorough digestion are also fundamental tenets of the Mayr diet. This entails taking your time with each mouthful and thoroughly chewing your food to fully appreciate it. For optimal digestion and nutrient absorption, food must be thoroughly chewed.

• The Mayr diet stresses the significance of combining ingredients properly. To achieve this, you must combine certain substances and avoid others.

It cautions against consuming protein and carbohydrates at the same meal, as this can make digestion more difficult. Instead, the diet recommends pairing carbohydrates with vegetables or healthful fats, and proteins with non-starchy vegetables.

• Frequently, the Mayr diet incorporates fasting or calorie restriction. Intermittent fasting, in which you alternate between periods of fasting and eating, and protracted fasting are viable options. Some individuals believe that fasting can assist them in losing weight, cleansing their bodies, and rejuvenating their digestive systems.

It is important to note that patients and doctors may interpret the Mayr Diet differently. In many instances, the diet is merely one component of a comprehensive Mayr Therapy program that also includes abdominal massages, hydrotherapy, and individualized treatment plans.

Before commencing a new diet or wellness program, you should always consult your doctor or a registered dietitian to ensure that it will help you achieve your specific health goals.

CHAPTER TWO

Preparing To Commence The Mayr Diet

If you take the time to prepare for the Mayr Diet, you will be able to make a seamless transition and reap the most benefits from it. Consider the following advice.

• Do your research and learn as much as possible about the Mayr diet and how it operates. Read books, articles, or consult credible sources to learn more about the theory, acceptable foods, and best practices. With this knowledge, you can set reasonable objectives and mentally prepare.

• Prior to commencing any new diet or wellness program, it is recommended that you consult a healthcare professional, such as a registered dietitian or a physician familiar with the Mayr Diet. They are qualified to evaluate your specific health conditions, determine if the diet is secure for you, and provide you with individualized recommendations.

• You should purge your pantry of processed foods, refined carbohydrates, and any other potential triggers. You should stock up on fruits, vegetables, lean meats, whole grains, and healthful fats, among other whole, unprocessed foods.

• Keeping a well-stocked pantry with Mayr-approved foods can make it easier to adhere to the diet.

• To save time and money, make an effort to organize your meals in advance. Create a menu that adheres to the Mayr Diet guidelines and includes a variety of nutrient-rich foods.

This will allow you to keep your week more organized and choose healthier options. If you want to save time and ensure that you always have nutritious food on hand, consider batch cooking and meal planning.

• Mindfulness practices during meals are central to the Mayr diet. Learn to savor each morsel and focus on what you are doing while eating. Do not consume food or watch television while distracted. Learn to pay attention to your body's requirements and eat accordingly.

• Depending on your current eating habits, it may be preferable to implement the Mayr Diet progressively as opposed to making sudden, drastic changes. Eliminate allergen-causing foods one by one and introduce Mayr-recommended alternatives progressively. The transition to the new dietary recommendations should be less difficult if you take things slowly.

• Seek out a friend or community member who is also on the Mayr Diet or who has experience with it for advice and motivation.

Sharing your experiences, gaining knowledge from others, and having someone hold you accountable can make it easier to motivate yourself and overcome obstacles along the path.

Keep in mind that the Mayr Diet is only one component of the Mayr Method, which addresses numerous health and digestion concerns.

Changing one's diet should be considered in the context of a person's overall health, and professional advice should be sought for personalized recommendations.

Homewares And Cooking Utensils For The Kitchen

Investing in high-quality kitchen equipment and materials will make meal preparation and cooking enjoyable. While preferences differ, the following appliances and supplies are common in most homes:

1. Equipment for the kitchen:

• Variable-sized nonstick, stainless steel, and cast-iron pots and pans.

• Baking dishes and platters.

• Ovenware dish.

• Crock cooker or Dutch oven.

• Saucier.

2. Cooking utensils:

• Knife for culinary use.

• The Knife for Paring.

• Cooking knife.

- Knife snips.

- Wooden spoons.

- Metal or silicone spatulas.

- Stir.

- Pliers.

- Spatula.

- Spoons and measuring glasses.

- An implement for opening tinned food.

- Peeler for vegetable preparation.

3. Home appliances:

- Oven.

- Cooktop and oven.

• Microwave oven.

• Blending device.

• Cooking equipment;.

• Toasting appliance/oven.

• The electric tea kettle.

• Espresso or coffee equipment.

• Crockpot or alternative slow cooker.

• Electric or manual mixers, or both.

4. Utensils for cooking:

• Mixing bowls in a variety of sizes.

• Baking utensils.

• Cake pans.

• Muffin and cupcake pans.

• Bread fungus.

• A shaping pin.

• Cooler container.

5. Kitchen Aids:

• Either an analog or digital thermometer.

• Kitchen Balance.

• Shredder.

• Citrus juicer.

• Garlic press.

• Strainer or sieve.

• Spinner for salad preparation.

• A mandoline for dicing.

• Peeling tool.

6. Containers for Storing Items:

• Plastic containers and additional food storage products.

• Glass canisters, such as Mason jars.

• To preserve delicacies, wrap them in plastic, aluminum foil, or parchment paper.

• There are Ziploc containers.

7. Not specified:

• Spoons used for mixing.

- Towels or oven mittens for cooking.

- Dishrags and Towels.

- Apparel.

- Containers for dry products, such as jars and canisters.

- Containers for the storage or presentation of seasonings.

- Oil or conditioner for cutting surfaces (if wood is utilized).

Keep in mind that this is merely a starting point, and that your actual needs may vary depending on your cooking manner, preferences, and menu plans. It is prudent to assess your culinary needs and augment your supply of essentials over time.

Food And Meal Planning Diaries

Planning meals in advance and maintaining a food journal can facilitate the maintenance of a well-organized and healthy diet. Each is summarized in the following sections.

Meal planning is the process of organizing one's food consumption for a specific period of time, typically a week, in advance. The potential benefits include the following:

• By planning one's meals for the week and then creating a purchasing list based on the ingredients needed, one can save both time and money. In addition to reducing food waste, you can save time by doing so.

• When you have a plan, it is simpler to prepare meals that are well-thought-out and nutritionally sound. Dietary needs or inclinations can be met by incorporating nutrient-dense foods and a balance of macronutrients (carbohydrates, proteins, and fats).

• Meal preparation can help you avoid overeating by promoting mindful dining and portion control. By increasing one's awareness of what and how much they consume, mindful eating is promoted.

• When you have a plan in place, you are relieved of the burden of deciding what to cook each day. Meal planning can reduce stress because it provides structure and reduces decision fatigue.

Instructions for preparing meals:

• Each week, you should designate time for meal planning and grocery shopping.

• Plan your meals around your active days, and prepare simpler meals on days with less activity.

• Each meal should include lean protein, complex carbohydrates, fiber-rich fruits and vegetables, and heart-healthy lipids.

• To save time during the week when preparing, wash and chop vegetables in advance.

• Experiment with cooking in bulk and leftovers to save time and always have nutritious meals on hand.

Through the use of a food journal, you can keep track of everything you consume throughout the day. It is a helpful tool for monitoring your food intake, identifying trends, and identifying problem areas.

Keeping a food journal can be beneficial in numerous ways.

• Accountability and self-awareness: keeping track of what you consume can help you become more aware of your eating patterns and better comprehend how you may be falling short of your nutritional goals.

• Diet adherence, weight loss, and the management of food allergies and intolerances are a few of the objectives that can be monitored with the aid of a food diary.

• Keeping note of what you consume can help you determine what triggers your digestive issues, food allergies, and emotional eating. The findings may also cast light on habits such as mindless eating and the relationship between what you consume and your mood.

Tips for recording your diet:

• Maintain a detailed food and drink journal, documenting serving sizes, preparation methods, and additional ingredients.

- Maintain a food journal using a notebook, an app, or a website.

- Inputs should as closely reflect reality as feasible. Please specify ingredients and preparation instructions if possible.

- While eating, be mindful of the day and time, your level of hunger, your emotions, and the events in your life.

- Regularly assess your eating behaviors to identify patterns and make adjustments.

- You should keep in mind that both meal planning and keeping a food journal are adaptable strategies that can be tailored to your requirements and preferences. They are designed to help you achieve your health and fitness goals while also promoting more mindful consumption and a more balanced diet land.

CHAPTER THREE
Phase 1 Detoxification Of The Mayr Diet

The first phase of the Mayr diet is also referred to as the "Detoxification" phase. It is intended to purge the body of toxins, reduce inflammation, and assist digestion. Here are some of this era's most prominent characteristics:

• Foods that may be difficult to digest or that induce inflammation should be avoided or significantly reduced during the Detoxification phase. This category may include certain additives or preservatives, processed foods, refined carbohydrates, gluten, dairy products, caffeine, and alcohol.

• Foods that are gentle on the digestive system are strongly suggested. To achieve this, many individuals consume more soups, herbal beverages, steamed or poached vegetables and fish. Whole grains and other foods abundant in fiber could also be included.

• The Detoxification phase emphasizes the significance of eating mindfully and thoroughly chewing food. Eating slowly and chewing food thoroughly can facilitate digestion and nutrient absorption.

• Maintaining a healthy fluid intake is essential at this time. Consuming large amounts of water and herbal infusions throughout the day facilitates detoxification by flushing out toxins.

• During the Detoxification phase, techniques to facilitate elimination and encourage regular gastrointestinal movements may be utilized. Doctors may recommend herbal supplements, natural laxatives, and mild abdominal massages.

- The Detoxification phase of the Mayr Diet is frequently performed under the supervision of a medical professional or as part of a formalized Mayr Therapy program. They can tailor recommendations to your unique requirements, monitor your progress, and ensure that any dietary changes are beneficial and healthy.

- Detoxification periods can be brief or lengthy, depending on the individual and their goals. To ensure that this step is suitable for your health and nutritional requirements, it is best to consult a medical professional and incorporate it into a larger wellness plan.

Please bear in mind that despite the growing popularity of the Mayr Diet and its numerous variations, there is a dearth of solid scientific evidence to support its claims. Before making significant dietary alterations, it is prudent to consult a physician or a qualified dietician.

Phase 2 Of The Mayr Diet: Gut Healing

Phase 2 of the Mayr Diet is commonly referred to as the "Gut Restoration" phase. During this phase, the stomach is treated to restore health, digestion is improved, and a healthy microbiota is nurtured. Here are some of this era's most prominent characteristics:

• During the Gut Restoration phase, a wider variety of foods are reintroduced, with an emphasis on those that are known to be gut-friendly.

Probiotics found in sauerkraut, kimchi, kefir, and yogurt help maintain a healthy microbiota in the digestive tract. Onions, garlic, leeks, asparagus, and oats are examples of prebiotic-rich foods that can be incorporated because they nourish beneficial microorganisms in the digestive tract.

• Fibre is emphasized because it is essential for digestive health. Whole grains, legumes, fruits, and vegetables are among the fiber-rich foods that should be ingested during this time. These are advantageous because they nourish the microorganisms in the gut and encourage regular bowel motions.

• The Mayr diet stresses the importance of combining foods in a manner that facilitates digestion. Eating large quantities of raw and cooked foods and concentrating on meals with a combination of macronutrients are examples of how to achieve this objective.

• The importance of thoroughly chewing food and consuming mindfully is emphasized during the Gut Restoration stage. This facilitates digestion and nutrient assimilation by breaking down food particles.

• Maintaining hydration, particularly with soothing fluids, is essential for colon health. Regular consumption of water and herbal teas promotes general health and assists digestion.

• Professional guidance, such as that of a physician or a qualified dietitian conversant with the Mayr Method, is strongly recommended for the duration of the Mayr Diet. In order to ensure that the dietary changes you make have a positive effect on your health, they can tailor their advice to your specific requirements and objectives.

Individual circumstances and intended results will determine the duration of the Gut Restoration phase. As part of a larger wellness plan, it is advisable to seek professional assistance for this step.

Before making significant dietary changes or beginning a new eating plan, you should always consult your physician or a registered dietitian. They can tailor their recommendations to your unique health needs and assist you in making informed decisions.

The Third Phase Of The Mayr Diet: Sustaining Results

"Long-Term Maintenance" is a prevalent name for Phase 3 of the Mayr Diet. This stage entails incorporating flexibility and balance into your long-term eating plan, as well as maintaining the healthy behaviors and dietary changes attained in earlier stages. Among the defining characteristics of this era are the following:

• Long-term maintenance necessitates an individualized approach, given that individuals have diverse nutritional needs and preferences. It suggests tailoring the diet to the individual's unique requirements, preferences, and health objectives.

• Mindful and intuitive eating: Maintaining your mindfulness practice around food is essential at the moment. You can maintain a healthy relationship with food if you pay attention to your body's signals of appetite and fullness and observe how it reacts to the different meals you consume.

• Meals that are both nutrient-dense and varied: this aspect cannot be overlooked. Fruits, vegetables, whole grains, lean meats, and healthy fats are examples of nutrient-dense foods that can help you meet your nutritional requirements and maintain your health.

• Moderation and flexibility: the Long-Term Maintenance phase encourages a more relaxed eating style by permitting the occasional consumption of munchies and extra calories. It advocates moderation over strict restriction.

• It is essential to maintain a healthy level of hydration during the Long-Term Maintenance phase. Digestion and general health can both benefit from consuming plenty of water and other hydrating fluids like herbal teas or infused waters.

• This phase emphasizes body awareness and self-care as dietary modifications are made. Optimizing your health can be as straightforward as observing how different foods affect your mood and adjusting your diet accordingly.

- Seeking sustained support from a healthcare practitioner, registered dietitian, or wellness coach can be beneficial, even though the Long-Term Maintenance phase is less structured than the other phases. You can rely on them for guidance, have them monitor your progress, and obtain solutions to any issues that arise.

In the Long-Term Maintenance phase, you will focus on developing lifelong healthy eating practices.

Always consult your physician or a qualified dietitian for personalized nutritional advice, as everyone has slightly different nutritional needs and preferences.

The Mayr Diet is only one of many conceivable diets, and there is little evidence to support its claims about how it works or how long it takes to produce results. Before making any health-related decisions, you should always conduct research and consult with experts who can modify their advice to your unique situation.

CHAPTER FOUR
Utilizing The Mayr Diet

To enhance digestion, gastrointestinal health, and overall health, the Mayr Diet must be implemented according to its principles and guidelines. The following are instructions for initiating the Mayr Diet:

• Familiarize yourself with the Mayr Diet's tenets and guidelines. Learn why it's so important to prioritize mindful dining, thorough chewing, food mixing, and protecting your digestive system.

• Speak with a specialist, such as a physician, registered dietitian, or

Mayr practitioner, who can tailor recommendations to your unique health situation and desired outcomes. They can tailor the Mayr diet to your specific requirements.

• The Mayr Diet is typically implemented in stages, including cleansing, gastrointestinal healing, and maintenance. Consult your physician to determine the duration of each stage and the rate at which you should progress through them.

• Preparation is the key to success when it comes to the Mayr diet's meal planning. Consume an abundance of fresh vegetables, lean proteins, and healthy lipids, and avoid processed foods whenever possible. Consider the proper method to combine foods, such as avoiding starch with protein.

•   Mindful eating involves concentrating on what you are consuming, slowing down, and chewing each bite thoroughly. Try chewing each mouthful a minimum of 20 to 30 times to improve digestion and increase sensations of fullness.

• Adequate hydration necessitates consistent water consumption throughout the day. Herbal beverages and infusions can promote digestion and hydration.

- Gut-friendly foods should be progressively introduced during the Gut Restoration stage. These include fermented foods (like sauerkraut and kefir) and foods abundant in prebiotics (like onions, garlic, and oats). These foods may help maintain a healthy gut microbiota.

- After completing the initial phases of the Mayr Diet, you should concentrate on maintaining the healthy habits and guiding principles that got you this far. Prioritize moderation, balance, and variety in your diet.

• Schedule follow-up appointments with your doctor or a registered dietitian to discuss your progress, any difficulties you're experiencing, and any dietary adjustments that may be necessary.

• Observe how your body reacts to various foods and make dietary adjustments as necessary. Due to the fact that everyone has distinct needs, it is essential to pay attention to your body's signals and make adjustments accordingly.

It is essential to remember that the Mayr Diet is just one of many options, and that the scientific community may not concur with its exact principles or purported benefits.

When it comes to your health, it is essential to conduct research, pay attention to your body, and consult with professionals who can modify their advice to your specific situation.

Dietary Schedule And Recipes For The Initial Phase Of Detoxification

During the Detoxification phase of the Mayr Diet, it is essential to consume foods that are low in potential triggers and high in moderate, easily digestible foods. Below are listed recipes and a sample detox diet plan.

Please note that this is merely an example, and your meal plan should be tailored to your specific dietary needs and preferences. If you desire individualized advice, consulting a physician or dietitian is recommended.

Here is an Illustration of a Detox Diet:

Breakfast consists of:

• Warm water with half a squeezed lemon is an excellent way to start the day.

• For "soft-cooked" eggs, the shells must be firm while the yolks must be runny.

• Steamed vegetables such as broccoli, cauliflower, and zucchini are delectable.

• Herbal teas: decompress with a cup of peppermint or chamomile tea.

The lunch menu:

• For a delicious salad of mixed greens, combine several varieties of salad greens, cucumber, radishes, and a light vinaigrette dressing of olive oil and lemon juice.

• Poached or steamed fish, such as salmon or cod: Prepare a dish.

• Asparagus steamed until crisp-tender; an excellent side dish option.

• Herbal tea or water: To stay hydrated, consume herbal tea or water.

The snack is:

• Fresh fruit: apple slices, melon cubes, and cherries.

Dinner is:

• Vegetable soup: prepare your own vegetable broth using an assortment of fresh vegetables, including carrots, celery, onions, and greens. Prepare a soup or stew with herbs and seasonings using vegetable stock or water as the base.

• Grill a chicken breast until it is fully cooked, then serve it with the vegetable broth.

• Greens, such as spinach or kale, can be steamed as a side dish and then gently seasoned with lemon juice.

• Herbal tea and water: Consume herbal tea and water.

A Snack Prior to Bed:

• Unwind with a cup of medicinal chamomile or lavender tea.

• Throughout the Detoxification phase, you should consume predominantly unprocessed foods. Avoid refined foods, coffee, alcoholic beverages, and added sugars.

Recipes to Try Throughout the Detoxification Process:

Steamed Fish Flavored with Lemon and Herbs:

• Season a piece of fish (such as cod or tilapia) with lemon juice, salt, and your favorite herbs (dill or parsley work well).

• Steam the fish for several minutes in a sterilizer.

• If desired, include a serving of steamed greens.

2. Green Smoothie for Cleansing:

• Combine one cup of coconut water with a fistful of spinach or kale, half a cucumber, a piece of ginger, one lemon's juice, and the remaining lemon.

• If preferred, a small apple or pear can be added for sweetness.

• Blend and consume as a nutritious and tasty smoothie.

3. Salad containing heated quinoa:

• Prepare quinoa according to the package's instructions.

• In a skillet, sauté diced bell peppers, zucchini, and cherry tomatoes in olive oil.

• Season the cooked quinoa with salt, pepper, and a splash of lemon juice before incorporating the sautéed vegetables.

• Serve warm as a nutritious and refreshing salad.

Taste frequently and modify ingredients and serving sizes

accordingly. To ensure that the diet is appropriate for you and to receive individualized guidance during the Detoxification process, it is best to consult a physician or registered dietitian.

The Gut Restoration phase of the Mayr Diet is characterized by the reintroduction of a wider variety of foods while prioritizing gut-friendly choices and appropriate food pairing. Below are recipe ideas and a sample menu for the Gut Restoration phase.

Please note that this is merely an example, and your meal plan should be tailored to your specific dietary needs and preferences. If you desire individualized advice, consulting a physician or dietitian is recommended.

Menu Designed to Restore Gut Health:

Breakfast consists of:

• Chia pudding can be prepared by combining chia seeds with unsweetened almond milk and refrigerating the mixture overnight. Serve with whipped cream and a sprinkling of chopped nuts.

• Water or herbal tea: Enjoy a glass of restorative water or herbal tea.

The lunch menu:

• Quinoa salad with caramelized vegetables. Prepare the quinoa and allow to settle. Several vegetables, including peppers, eggplant, and zucchini, taste fantastic when roasted. Serve the quinoa and roasted vegetables with a light vinaigrette made with olive oil and apple cider vinegar.

• To increase your protein intake, grill some chicken breasts or tofu.

• Herbal tea or water: To stay hydrated, consume herbal tea or water.

The snack is:

• A delectable and nutritious snack is Greek yogurt with fresh berries and a sprinkle of nuts or seeds.

Dinner is:

• Before baking, salmon fillets are seasoned with lemon juice, herbs (such as dill or thyme), salt, and pepper. Prepare well in the oven.

• Boil broccoli florets until crisp-tender, then sauté in a pan with olive oil and minced garlic.

• Salmon and steamed broccoli are served atop a bed of prepared quinoa or brown rice.

• Herbal tea and water: Consume herbal tea and water.

A Snack Prior to Bed:

• Smoothie that is gentle on the digestive system, made with coconut milk, frozen berries, spinach, almond butter, and cinnamon.

Try These Recipes While Your Gut Heals:

1. Bone broth for gastrointestinal health:

• For the best broth, simmer beef or poultry bones in water with aromatics such as bay leaves and thyme for a considerable amount of time.

• After cooking the broth, strain it and consume it as a digestive-friendly beverage or use it as a soup or stew base.

2. Carrot and Ginger Soup for Gas Relief:

• We will first sauté the shallots, ginger, and garlic in olive oil to soften them.

• Peel and slice some carrots, then combine them with vegetable broth and a pinch of turmeric. Continue simmering the carrots until they are fork-tender.

• Blend until smooth after seasoning with salt, pepper, and a dash of lemon juice.

3. Healthy Fermented Vegetables for the Stomach:

• Select carrots, cucumbers, and cabbage.

• Once the vegetables have been sliced or shredded, place them in a receptacle.

• Season to suit with salt and spices. To enhance the flavor of vegetables, massage them.

Place the lid on the container and leave it at room temperature for several days to ferment. After fermentation, refrigerate and use as a condiment or salad addition.

Taste frequently and modify ingredients and serving sizes accordingly. Consult a physician or registered dietitian if you want to ensure that the diet plan is appropriate for you and that you will receive specific support during the Gut Restoration phase.

Recipes And Meal Plans For The Third And Final Phase Of Weight Loss

During the Long-Term Maintenance phase of the Mayr Diet, the emphasis is on maintaining healthful habits and consuming a balanced diet. The following is a sample menu for the Maintenance phase, along with dish suggestions:

Please note that this is merely an example, and your meal plan should be tailored to your specific dietary needs and preferences. If you desire individualized advice, consulting a physician or dietitian is recommended.

Example of a Meal Plan for Long-Term Maintenance:

Breakfast consists of:

• Prepare scrambled eggs with vegetables by combining eggs, milk, salt, and pepper. Cubed cooked vegetables, including shallots, bell peppers, and spinach. The eggs are scrambled by adding them to the pan.

• Scrambled eggs with whole grain toast is a classic brunch dish.

Eat some sliced watermelon or a bowl of berries as fresh produce.

• Herbal tea or water: first thing in the morning, consume herbal tea or water.

The lunch menu:

• Add a protein source, such as grilled chicken, chickpeas, or shrimp, to a dish of mixed greens, cherry tomatoes and cucumber.

• Add cooked quinoa or brown rice to the salad for additional protein and fiber.

Dress the salad with a mild vinaigrette, such as one prepared with olive oil, lemon juice, and herbs.

• Herbal tea or water: To stay hydrated, consume herbal tea or water.

The snack is:

• Greek yogurt with crushed nuts and seeds: For a delectable and nutritious snack, top a serving of Greek yogurt with crushed nuts, seeds (such as chia or flax), and a drizzle of honey or maple syrup.

Dinner is:

• Salmon fillets or tofu that have been perfectly marinated and grilled.

• For a delectable side dish, combine Brussels sprouts, sweet potatoes, and carrots and roast them with olive oil, herbs, and spices.

• Quinoa or cauliflower rice makes an excellent side dish for seared salmon or tofu.

• Herbal tea and water: Consume herbal tea and water.

A Snack Prior to Bed:

• Almonds, pumpkin seeds, and dried cranberries are just a few of the nuts, seeds, and fruits that can be used to create a healthy and delicious trail mix.

Recipes for the Maintenance Phase:

1. Herbed Roasted Chicken:

• Season the chicken with salt, pepper, and a mixture of herbs (including rosemary, thyme, and garlic powder).

• Place in the oven and bake until the fluids are transparent.

• Prepare quinoa or brown rice to accompany the steamed vegetables.

2. Bell Peppers Stuffed with Quinoa:

• The crowns, seeds, and membranes should be eliminated from bell peppers.

• Sauté diced vegetables (such as zucchini, mushrooms, or spinach) with minced garlic and onion.

• Combine the cooked quinoa with the vegetables that have been sautéed in olive oil, herbs, salt, and pepper.

• Bake the packed bell peppers until soft and the filling is hot.

3. Vegetable and Tofu Stir-Fry:

• Several colorful vegetables, including broccoli, bell peppers, carrots, and snap peas, can be sautéed in a hot pan with a touch of oil.

• Add cubed tofu and sauté it in a wok over high heat until it is lightly browned and the vegetables are still crisp-tender.

• Soy sauce, ginger, and garlic are all excellent seasonings.

• This dish pairs well with brown rice or cauliflower rice.

- Taste frequently and modify ingredients and portion sizes accordingly. It is suggested that you consult a physician or dietitian.

CHAPTER FIVE
Delicious And Healthy Mayr Diet Dishes

Certainly! Here are a few healthful and delicious recipes that adhere to the guidelines of the Mayr Diet:

1. Grilled Lemon-Herb Chicken:

• Chicken breasts should be marinated in a mixture of lemon juice, minced garlic, fresh herbs (such as rosemary, thyme, and parsley), salt, and pepper for at least 30 minutes.

• Grill the poultry until completely cooked, juicy, and charred on the exterior.

- Accompanied by quinoa or roasted sweet potatoes and steamed asparagus or green beans.

2. Quinoa salad with grilled vegetables.

- Using olive oil, salt, and pepper, roast a variety of vegetables, such as cherry tomatoes, bell peppers, zucchini, and red onions, until tender and slightly caramelized.

- Prepare quinoa according to the instructions on the package, then set aside to chill.

- In a bowl, combine the cooked quinoa, fresh herbs (such as basil or cilantro), lemon juice, and extra virgin olive oil with the roasted vegetables.

• Modify the seasonings as necessary and serve as a fresh salad.

3. Baked salmon with a dill dressing:

• Season salmon fillets with salt, pepper, and a dash of lemon juice.

• Bake the salmon in a preheated oven at 400 degrees Fahrenheit (200 degrees Celsius) for 12 to 15 minutes, or until it reaches the doneness you choose.

In a small bowl, combine Greek yogurt, fresh dill, lemon zest, minced garlic, salt, and pepper to create a creamy dill sauce.

• Serve the salmon with steamed broccoli or a salad of mixed greens and a dollop of dill sauce.

4. Green Smoothie for Cleansing:

• Blend together a small apple, some lemon juice, a splash of coconut water, and a fistful of spinach or kale until creamy.

• You can add chia seeds or protein powder for additional nourishment.

• Combine all ingredients and serve as a detoxifying smoothie.

5. Soup Including Digestive-Healing Vegetables:

• Sauté diced onions, carrots, and celery in olive oil in a large saucepan until they are tender.

• Cook the garlic, ginger, and turmeric for one minute, or until the fragrances of the garlic and ginger are released.

• Bring vegetable broth to a simmer, then add it to the dish. Add some chopped vegetables, such as broccoli, cauliflower, or verdant greens.

• Cook the greens at a moderate simmer until they are fork-tender. Add seasonings such as salt, pepper, and perhaps fresh herbs such as parsley or cilantro.

• The vegetable soup should be served heated, along with a dollop of Greek yogurt and a few squeezes of lemon juice.

• Don't neglect to adjust the serving sizes and ingredients to suit your preferences and dietary restrictions. To add variety and flavor to your Mayr Diet dishes, try experimenting with new herbs, seasonings, and vegetables. Savor your cuisine and recognize its nutritional value.

Adapting To A New Lifestyle

The Mayr Diet has a greater impact on health and well-being when combined with other healthy lifestyle changes. The following adjustments to your daily regimen are suggested:

• To complement the Mayr Diet and enhance your overall health, incorporate regular exercise into your daily routine. If these activities interest you, walk, cycle, ride a bike, swim, and practice yoga. Aim for at least 75 minutes per week of intense exercise or 150 minutes per week of moderate exercise.

• Techniques for managing stress include deep breathing, meditation, yoga, and finding enjoyable activities that allow you to temporarily divert your attention from your concerns. Understanding how to manage stress in a healthy manner is crucial for maintaining good digestive health if you are a chronic stress sufferer.

• Make getting a decent night's sleep a priority every night; most adults should aim for seven to nine hours. Getting sufficient, high-quality sleep improves the health of the digestive system. Establish a routine of going to bed at the same time every night and making your bedroom conducive to slumber.

• Consume copious amounts of water throughout the day to keep your body hydrated. Your digestive tract and other internal processes can both benefit from consuming plenty of water. Aim for at least eight cups (64 ounces) of water per day, but consume more if you're very active or in a hot environment.

• Mindful eating involves recognizing when one is hungry and when one is satisfied. Focus on the flavors and textures of the food, and chew each morsel thoroughly. As a result, your digestive system will improve, you will consume less food, and you will have a more positive attitude toward food.

• Limit your consumption of processed foods and added carbohydrates because they are likely to be high in unhealthy fats, sugar, and synthetic chemicals. Instead, you should consume digestive tract-friendly, nutrient-dense, unprocessed, whole meals.

• Plan your meals to include an assortment of fruits, vegetables, whole grains, and lean proteins, as well as a balance of macronutrients (carbohydrates, proteins, and healthy lipids). This protects your digestive health by supplying a vast array of nutrients.

• Assemble a group of supporters, including friends, family, and neighbors, who support and believe in your efforts to improve your health. Having people cheer you on and hold you accountable can be a tremendous motivational lift.

Remember that incorporating lifestyle changes takes time and fortitude. It is essential to implement changes that are both manageable and beneficial in the long term. Before making significant adjustments to your diet or daily routine, it is best to consult a doctor or certified dietitian for individualized recommendations based on your needs and health condition.

CHAPTER SIX
Methods Of Stress Management

Managing tension is crucial to maintaining good health. Listed below are some easy-to-implement strategies for managing tension.

• By practicing deep breathing exercises, relaxation and tension reduction can be enhanced. Find a spot where you won't be disturbed to sit or slumber. Inhale deeply through the nostrils and exhale entirely through the mouth.

• Pay close attention to your respiration and observe the rise and fall of your abdomen as you take deep breaths in and out. When you feel apprehensive or overwhelmed, focus on your breathing for a few minutes.

• Meditation is an effective way to reduce stress and calm the psyche. Find a tranquil area and reside there. Try closing your eyes and focusing on your respiration or another activity. Don't attempt to control your thoughts; just let them come and go. Meditation should be pursued gradually and persistently over time.

• Mindfulness entails paying attention to the present moment without formulating judgments about what is observed.

- Practice being present during mundane activities such as dining, walking, and washing dishes. Focus on being aware of your perceptions, ideas, and emotions without becoming attached to them. This activity has the capacity to alleviate both tension and a lack of self-awareness.

- Regular exercise is one of the most effective methods for combating tension. Endorphins are the compounds that are released during vigorous exercise. If walking, jogging, dancing, or yoga interest you, engage in these activities. On most days of the week, 30 minutes of physical activity is recommended.

• Effective time management may help you feel less hurried and more in control of your day. Create a schedule or a list of tasks and prioritize them by importance. Establish goals that are attainable and designate time for rest and self-care.

• Communicate with your social network for much-needed morale enhancement. Stress can be reduced by communicating with a trusted individual. Make an effort to meet new people and engage in group activities to facilitate friendship formation.

• Experiment with different relaxation techniques until you find one that works for you. Try aromatherapy with essential oils, take a warm bath, practice yoga or tai chi, engage in some of your favorite pastimes, or make something new.

• Healthy lifestyle habits may help you cope with stress in a constructive manner. Maintaining a healthy lifestyle involves the fundamentals of getting enough sleep, eating well, limiting coffee and alcohol consumption, and consuming enough water. It has been demonstrated that maintaining excellent physical health increases stress resistance.

Keep in mind that everyone has different requirements when it comes to managing stress. Discover what resonates with you and incorporate it into your daily existence. Seek the assistance of a mental health professional or therapist if you are having difficulty managing tension on your own.

Get Some Quality Sleep And Rest

A decent night's sleep is irreplaceable for optimal health and stress management. Consider the following suggestions to maximize the benefits of your sleep and make it more restorative.

• Establish a consistent sleep schedule by going to bed and waking up at the same time every day, even on vacations. This improves the quality of your sleep and assists in resetting your body's internal rhythm.

• Transform your bedroom into a tranquil retreat where you can unwind and sleep. Maintain a cool, quiet, and dark atmosphere in your chamber. Make sure your mattress and pillows are supportive and comfortable, and install draperies or blinds to block out unwanted light and sound.

• Establish a Nightly Ritual: Do something relaxing before bed to signal to your body that it is time to settle down and prepare for sleep.

Reading a book, having a hot bath, performing some light stretching or yoga, or listening to soothing music are examples of this type of relaxation. Before slumber, avoid engaging in stimulating activities or using electronic devices with bright screens.

• Caffeine and alcohol consumption should be limited, and neither should be consumed after work. Both medications have the potential to alter your sleep schedule and diminish sleep quality.

• Avoid consuming large amounts of fluids, spicy or acidic foods, and heavy meals prior to bedtime, as these may cause discomfort and prohibit you from falling asleep. If you are hungry or thirsty, it is recommended to consume small snacks and sips of water.

• Reduce your tension before bedtime by reading a calming book or listening to calming music. Such activities include deep breathing exercises, maintaining a gratitude journal, meditating, and progressive muscle relaxation.

• Make your bedroom a tranquil, restful place to unwind before bedtime. Keep it clutter-free, don cozy pajamas and bedding, and consider using aromatherapy with calming scents such as lavender to decompress at the end of the day.

• Maintain a consistent exercise regimen to enhance your sleep hygiene and circadian rhythm.

However, vigorous exercise in the hours preceding bedtime may disrupt sleep.

• Reduce your screen time in the hours preceding bedtime. This includes television, mobile devices, and laptops. The blue light emitted by these devices has been shown to interfere with the body's natural melatonin production.

• Consult a Healthcare expert or Sleep Specialist: If you regularly have trouble sleeping or suspect you have a sleep disorder, it may be beneficial to consult a healthcare expert or sleep specialist.

Keep in mind that the quantity and quality of your sleep is directly related to your health and wellbeing. Sleep and refreshment should be your top priority when considering how to take care of yourself.

CHAPTER SEVEN
Movement And Exercise

Regular exercise and other forms of physical activity are necessary for good health. Prior to beginning an exercise regimen, it is essential to consider the following factors:

• Choose Entertaining Activities Seek out activities that appeal to your interests and are within your skill set. Physical activity includes walking, jogging, cycling, swimming, dancing, hiking, performing sports, and attending fitness classes. If you are enjoying yourself, you are more likely to persist.

• Ensure They're Realistic: Ensure that your objectives are SMART (specific, measurable, attainable, pertinent, and timely) and that you set a deadline for achieving them.

This will keep you motivated and allow you to track your progress. Create manageable short-term goals and work up to longer-term, more frequent goals.

• Increase the variety of your routines by incorporating exercises that target different muscle groups. This category includes strength training (with weights or resistance bands), cardio exercise (such as walking or cycling), flexibility training (such as yoga or stretching), and balance and coordination training (such as tai chi or Pilates).

• Consistency should be a top priority, so schedule daily or weekly exercise. To experience the long-term benefits of exercise, consistency is essential. Taking the stairs as opposed to the elevator and going for a brisk lunchtime stroll can both build up and make a difference.

• If you are new to exercise or returning after a period of inactivity, begin with low- to moderate-intensity activities and gradually increase the intensity as your fitness level improves. This is beneficial to your health and prevents injuries by allowing your body time to acclimate.

• Recognize Your Limits Pay attention to your body's cues and stay within your limits. If you experience pain, discomfort, or extreme fatigue while exercising, you should either slow down or cease and consult a doctor.

Warming up is the process of preparing your muscles for physical activity by undertaking dynamic stretching or low-intensity exercises. Similarly, a cool-down period consisting of light stretching can aid in recovery by enhancing flexibility.

• Drinking water before, during, and after exercise is sufficient for optimal hydration during exercise. This is notably true for extended or strenuous exercise sessions.

• Rest and recuperation time is essential, so be sure to allow for it. This promotes muscle growth and regeneration and protects against overuse issues. You should pay attention to your body's requirements, alternate the types of activities you perform, and schedule rest days.

- Consider meeting with a fitness expert, such as a personal trainer or exercise physiologist, if you are new to exercising, have special health concerns, or wish to enhance your fitness regimen. They will be able to provide you with specific advice, ensure that you are following an appropriate program, and maintain your physical fitness.

It is essential to remember that exercise should not feel like a burden. Find activities that fit into your schedule, and make it a habit to prioritize physical activity.

Resolving Problems And Making Progress

It is normal to encounter obstacles when attempting to establish a new routine, such as the Mayr Diet or an exercise regimen. Here are some of the most prevalent problems and their respective solutions:

• If you're having difficulty initiating your change, remind yourself of why you wanted to make it in the first place. Create well-defined objectives and frequently revisit them to maintain concentration. Make the transition to your new routine as enjoyable as possible by engaging in activities you appreciate, such as listening to music or a podcast while you exercise or experimenting with Mayr Diet foods.

• Busy schedules make it difficult to incorporate healthful behaviors such as cooking and exercise. Make room in your hectic agenda for these healthy activities.

Try to squeeze in little periods of exercise or meal preparation whenever possible during the day, whether that's first thing in the morning, during your lunch break, or after work. Additionally, preparing meals and doing dishes in abundance may save you time in the kitchen.

• Change is more difficult without the support of family and acquaintances. Inform your loved ones of your plans and the significance of your new lifestyle. Join an offline or online support group comprised of individuals who can relate to your situation and offer words of encouragement.

• It is normal for your health journey's progress to occasionally halt or even regress. If you have reached a weight loss or fitness plateau, it is time to reevaluate your approach and make adjustments.

If you require specific advice, consult your physician or a qualified nutritionist. Remember that delays are inevitable, but you should not abandon your objectives because of them.

• Food demands and temptation may make it difficult to adhere to the Mayr diet. Learn to consume mindfully and replace unhealthy foods with healthier alternatives. Remove unhealthy foods from view and stock up on healthy alternatives. Try new seasonings, spices, and cooking techniques to enhance the flavor and variety of your dishes.

• Emotional nutrition is a significant factor in failure. Try various means of coping with your emotions, such as meditation or yoga, speaking with trusted individuals, or expressing yourself creatively. The causes of emotional appetite can be addressed through journaling or therapy.

• Stop and reevaluate your methods if you feel as though you are making no progress. While following the Mayr Diet, you should consult a physician or a registered dietitian to ensure you are on the right course. Ensure that you are getting the most out of your exercises by monitoring your fitness level and level of difficulty.

It is essential to remember that changing your routine takes effort. Be compassionate to yourself and remember to celebrate your victories, no matter how minor. Maintain a growth mindset as opposed to a perfectionism mindset, and be adaptable in your approach. Remember that each day is an opportunity to recommit to your health and happiness, and seek assistance when necessary.

The Conclusion

Finally, the Mayr Diet is an all-inclusive program for improving your digestive and overall health. This strategy includes mindful dining, eating in the proper combinations, and consuming whole, unprocessed meals. Typical phases of a diet include detoxification, intestinal healing, and maintenance.

A successful implementation of the Mayr Diet requires preparation in the form of acquiring the necessary kitchen apparatus, supplies, and meal-planning tools. A food journal can be a useful tool for tracking progress and identifying areas for improvement.

Follow the phase-specific meal plans and recipes of the Mayr Diet to ensure that your body receives the nutrients it requires. These dishes should incorporate fruits, vegetables, whole grains, lean proteins, and healthy fats.

In addition to the nutritional component, the efficacy of the Mayr Diet can be enhanced in multiple ways. Eating mindfully, engaging in regular physical activity, obtaining sufficient rest, and other stress-reduction techniques all contribute significantly to one's health and contentment.

When making lifestyle changes, it is crucial to be patient and adaptable. With the assistance of healthcare professionals or registered dietitians, you can overcome obstacles and reach your objectives.

Keep in mind that the Mayr Diet is just one method for promoting digestive health, and that your results may vary based on how you implement it. Before making any significant dietary changes, particularly if you have certain health conditions or dietary restrictions, it is always advisable to consult with a qualified healthcare professional or dietitian.

Adopting the Mayr Diet's tenets and making modest, long-lasting adjustments to your lifestyle can improve your digestive health, enhance your overall well-being, and help you develop healthy habits for life.

THE END

www.ingramcontent.com/pod-product-compliance
Lightning Source LLC
Chambersburg PA
CBHW050732260726
48661CB00001B/199